DEDICATION

I dedicate this book to my family, without you I always feel empty and alone.

TABLE OF CONTENTS

Chapter 1 - Introduction to Extreme Weight Loss

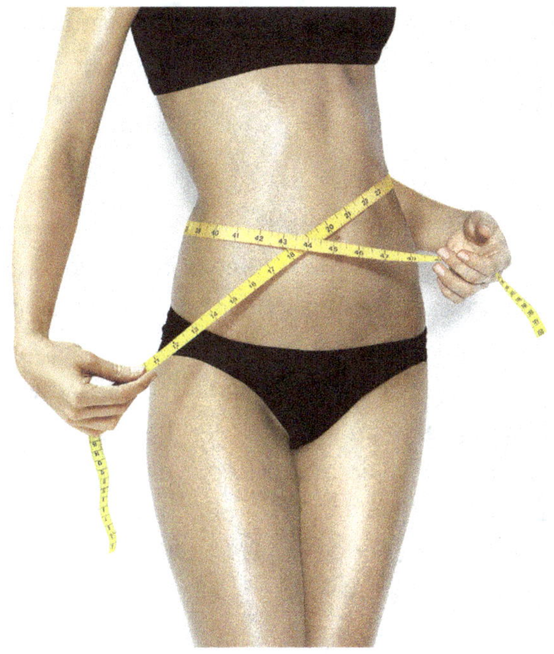

Publications are the first thing that authorities produce in order for them to effectively send their important message to the public; to be healthy with the help of Weight Loss Management. They produce and continue to create tools that can easily help them reach people who are not aware of their situation.

Basic Information

These publications are also composed of information in relation to the foods and procedures that people can follow in order to promote healthier living. By doing this, there are a lot of people that will no longer be unconscious of what specific processes of Weight Loss Management are preferred for their needs.

Health care providers are one of the most trusted entities that will never hesitate to help people who are struggling while accomplishing Weight Loss Management. These people are being taught about new and innovated processes, which are simply to conduct and maintain, so that they can elevate the number of healthy people in their place. With the contribution of this particular system, health providers will no longer have problems implementing better systems for the beneficial concerns of everyone.

Community groups and organizations that need support for the betterment of Weight Loss Management in the world also receive help that will educate them about what process of this healthy approach is necessary for each and every case or situation. In fact, these entities that work for the promotion of disease and illness-free societies help each other to attain the most positive results that they can achieve in accordance to Weight Loss Management. As long as community groups and organizations have the complete support and maintenance that they need, there is no way that they will not grant the desires of patients who look forward to brighter results in relation to their difficulties.

Pertaining to the focus and dedication of people who are not stopping in conquering and overcoming the cause and effect of Weight Loss Mismanagement, people who are now continuing to exert their best effort will no longer have difficulty in attaining the most recommend results that they've always wanted. By the time that they achieve these outcomes, they can now be more positive in their life perspectives which are the main reason of why they can be productive as a healthy human being.

Chapter 2- Importance of Setting Goals – Weight Loss Management

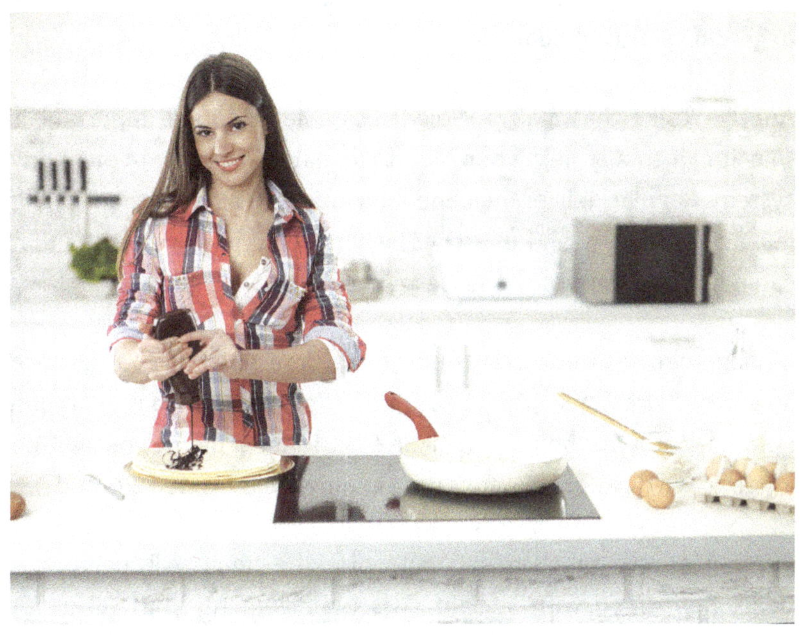

The significance of Weight Loss Management is now said to be the top priority of health providers and authorities. As health is a concern, there is a great possibility that a lot of people will now resolve their problems when the time comes now that they are conscious of how they will live healthier.

Performing each of these tasks consecutively will promote a chance for people to live longer and prosper at the same time. In accordance, it is better to know the following important facts about Weight Loss Management that will help you realize how valuable it is to possess.

Diabetes is considered to be one of the top illnesses possessed by younger and older individuals. As you know, diabetes generates a lot of difficulties for living if it is not prevented and treated properly. With the presence of Weight Loss Management, there is a definite chance that people can avoid the possibility of obtaining diabetes which can cause a lot of sickness' that are serious and incurable. Never neglect this type of condition if you have it because it can possibly make you weak as a person in terms of a degrading status of health.

Another thing that makes Weight Loss Management important is that it can totally help your blood circulate properly in your body system. Regular deliverance and circulation of blood, including the balance of its flow and existence, will develop positive results that can make you free from diseases and illnesses. Weight Loss

Management can also contribute to the presence of your glucose level that prevents your body from losing its strong immune system. With the help of Weight Loss Management, you will no longer have difficulty in generating healthy cells inside your body.

As long as you practice and patronize the healthy living that is being performed with Weight Loss Management, you will never lose your confidence as a person. A lot of obese individuals do not want to go out and have shop or do other activities because of their size and health condition. It is better to exercise so that you can maintain and prevent this kind of situation. Together with Weight Loss Management, you can now attain the confidence of being fit and suitable in everyday tasks and activities for the day.

Cholesterol, blood pressure, and any other type of cardiovascular disease can only be controlled and prevented by means of Weight Loss Management. Exercising everyday will give you more defenses against these illnesses that are considered to be some of the reasons why a person cannot properly accomplish all the tasks assigned to them for a day. Being unhealthy is not an option, especially when you have a family that is relying on the strength and confidence that can help you go through and through.

The Reason Goals Are Important

Weight reasons are commonly the reason to consider attaining a healthy and active life. With the contribution of a Weight Maintaining System, you will no longer have trouble in your plans as a person who targets a life that is suitable when facing different challenges of life, especially when it covers the existence of illnesses and diseases.

Weight Maintaining Systems

Weight Maintaining Systems will provide you with results that are and prouder to be promoted and suggested to other people. It is beneficial to achieve the outcomes that come from this system so that you can avoid the difficulty of obtaining a contented and happy life.

Calories in the body, if not balanced, can contribute weakness in to the body. Too much of anything is always bad and unhelpful. So whenever you possess an amount of calories that exceeds the capability of your body to restore, it is time to conduct a Weight Maintaining System. Maintaining your body weight as an average person can cut calories. A healthy and a balanced eating habit will help your diet objectives to become more successful and truly achievable.

Fiber helps the body system to operate properly. It also produces energy that can contribute to the betterment of your work which results in good accomplishments. A Weight Maintaining System is also important, considering the presence of fiber, since it is a factor that can eliminate the possibility of developing diseases. Fibers are also helpful in making a person fully conditioned every day. By the time that you attain this outcome coming from the existence of fiber, you will never have to worry about how you will maintain a great figure and weight.

A body that has a liquid composition which is balanced and clean is also important for the maintenance of your weight composition.

Water helps a person to feel full every now and then; as a result, they can now lose their appetite to eat which is unhealthy. Water is also beneficial for your digestive system because it will prevent the process of digestion from being difficult. Easy digestion helps the nutrients of the food reach every potential part of your body for the purpose of a strong and healthy life. Lastly, water it very valuable when it comes to the maintenance of the coolness and balanced hydration and perspiration system of your body.

Physical activity of the body will elevate your metabolism which is great for the productivity of your life. As a result, with the help of a Weight Maintaining System, you can now accomplish a lot of things that were incomparable before. In addition, it can also increase the rate of your metabolism which is considered to be a huge help for your body to resist diseases. Burning fat is now attainable in an effortless process.

Chapter 3- Body Image – Weight Loss Management

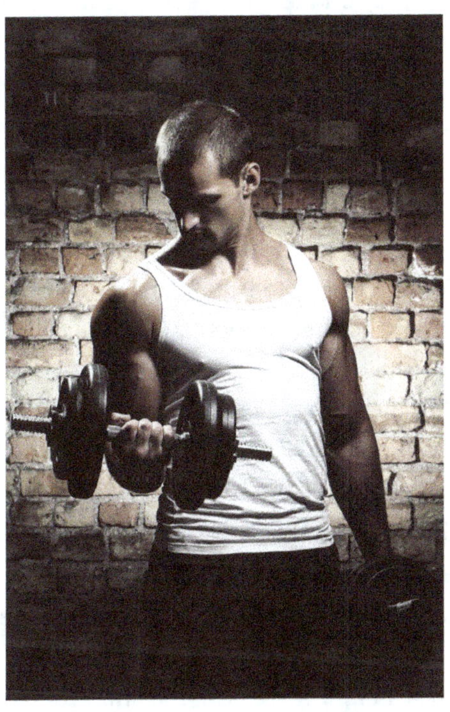

It's true that body image can really affect the way you live and tasks that you need to do for other people every day. Possessing good curves and muscles that are really strong will help a person execute better work and operations in their job because these factors will boost their confidence. It is also a fact that body image affects the impression of other people who are complete strangers. Together with a fit and healthy lifestyle, you can easily attain a body image that is commonly dreamed of by a lot of people.

Body Image Is Important

Having a good and proportioned body curve that is healthy at the same time will make you feel great every day. Since the function of body image is to expose your external beauty, people will evidently notice your responsible and truly disciplined way of living. Aside from these advantages, you can now attain the best confidence, self acceptance and self-worth which are really helpful for the development of your personality. You can also prevent tendencies that will lead you to eating habits and mood disorders that are really unhealthy for the reason that it can affect the psychological system of a person and they can become more depressed.

Your mind and body is always connected in every way, in this case, if you have a good body structure, there is a great chance that you can also have perspectives in life that are also good. So whenever people think that you possess a not so good fitness of body, it can also affect your mind, but never be disappointed about it, it is better to solve the problem with the help of a healthy and balanced diet with the accompaniment of regular exercise. This way of living will help you realize the importance of your body image.

Poor bodies might receive a lot of discrimination and other related insults that may cause a degrading effect to your confidence and self- esteem. It is good that you can accept the real you so that you will never feel insecure with other people who receive good impressions from the public. In this way, you can realize your worth as a person even if you are not perfect. It can also generate standards that will make you think more positive thoughts which deliver actions that are considered to be worth it and really satisfying as a well-being.

Valuing yourself is good things that can help an individual attain their plans for life. A healthy body promotes better thinking because it can provide you with thoughts that are stable enough for work and tasks which need immediate and contented solutions. Emotions and mental system that are stable will prevent you from conceptualizing things in life into negative ones. In this case, decreasing the probability of feeling depressed and the existence of anxieties is possible since these factors are the main reasons why a person thinks negatively of life.

Eating Right Key to Weight Loss

Eating balanced and healthy meals is one of the best ways a person can live longer and prosper. By the time you start living, specifically eating right, in a proper way, there is no way that you cannot feel great within yourself and in your outside appearance. A lot of beneficial effects are only possible when you start conducting this lifestyle. Never underestimate the power of this system and the food structure that composes this very healthy approach for it will definitely give you the assurance of obtaining a strong and positive well-being.

How to Eat Properly

Whole grains are one of the best types of food that are helpful for your plan in terms of eating right. Its abundance in the market can also contribute to your plan because you will never have difficulty finding these products. Another thing is that whole grains can be accompanied with different types of food like vegetables and fruits, and even milk; giving you a lot of options on how you can consume this food. The importance of whole grains in your body is that it can provide natural nutrients which are needed for the complete energy that is needed by your system every day. A variety of whole grain products can also make you more flexible on consuming these healthy foods.

Vegetables are already known for their beneficial effects on the body, but some people do not like to consume them because of their structure and appearance. This is the best thing about vegetables, because like fruits, they can now be drank by means of blending systems. Another thing that will amaze you with this food item is that it can be eaten raw. You just have to clean it properly. Placing vegetables in your plans of eating right can contribute to properly neutralizing the foods that you are consuming every day. It can also clean your body system because it has natural nutrients that cleanse your digestive system and other related factors.

Fruits are also considered a common food that is being consumed by people who want to have good eating habits. As you know, fruits are composed with different vitamins and minerals that create defenses for body to resist diseases and illnesses. They can also refresh the body to make it livelier. Fruits also serve as a natural tool that can make your skin more appealing and refreshed. As long as you consume fruits, there is no way that you cannot receive a natural approach to eating right.

Maintaining a diet that is composed of a low fat system is recognizable. If you are going to fry, just use non-stick pans so that you will no longer use oil that contains a lot of fats. Starting your morning with oatmeal, approximately one bowl, will give you the total benefits that are needed for the day. Limit your sweet food consumptions and avoid smoking. These are some of the particulars that can help you achieve your success in terms of eating right.

Chapter 4- Exercise Right to Extreme Weight Loss

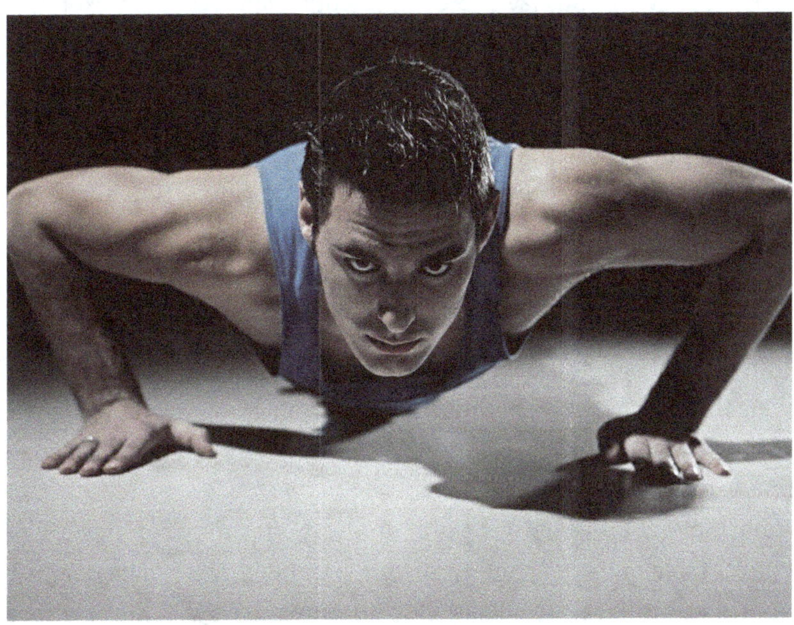

In order to achieve the effects from exercise that you desire, you must have motivation, dedication and discipline to maintain and obtain your target objectives. Yes it is difficult because you have a lot of commitments that are needed to be done every day. But since you want these things to be accomplished, you must consider making tackling these tasks in a healthy way.

Exercise Goal Pointers

It is always good for a particular body system to move and work precisely so that it can live healthy in any way possible. In order to achieve the best results from this plan, you have to focus on what your goals are and aim for them.

Specific goals are really important to be visualized as early as possible. This way you can prevent factors that can possibly affect your plans from being attained. Specific goals can also help you stay on the right track, as long as you stick to the plan, you will never be in a failing condition. You can also reduce the presence of reasons of why you have to change your plan regarding exercise. Maintaining yourself and remaining on the right track can give you the assurance of obtaining your plan and objectives.

Measurable goals are also significant to be realized. There is a great possibility of you being aware of your situation regarding your status of exercise when you know how to monitor your own operations. As long as you implement this kind of system, you will no longer have difficulty in controlling your eagerness that sometimes leads to accidents. Stopping yourself and not exceeding your body limit is a great advantage of maintaining a good balance of your body's capacity.

Adjustable goals are also helpful in a way that they can make you comfortable in the activities that you are doing. You can now adjust yourself in different challenges so that obstacles will never affect your lifestyle. This is a very effective system for exercising your body without having any injuries that come from unconditional tendencies. This process will also contribute to you being more flexible in every possible way. Since these goals are considered to be flexible, you can effortlessly change the route of your track without being lost.

An action-oriented goal refers to the application of exercises that cover your over-all plan in order to achieve your objectives for a healthy life.

In relation to realistic goals, this practice focuses on how you will implement serious and tough exercise programs that are really beneficial for a good body structure. Conducting and settling this goal will generate more power and motivation in your exercise.

Time-based goals are a specific plan that concentrates on your availability to do the exercise. Since you always a have a busy working schedule, it is a must that you set a day that will focus on your training which will never affect the process that you have to do within that day.

If you are done deciding to be healthy by means of preserving a body image that is truly beneficial for everyone, then your decision is really looking forward for a brighter future and perspective in life. As you know, being fit and sexy at the same time means a lot of opportunities and chances to be noticed not only your outside appearance, but also your well-disciplined personality that is commonly attained by successful people. Giving yourself multiple credits is now possible by working with this procedure of elevating the condition of your body's image.

Body Image Goals

Lasting relationship is achievable as long as you preserve your beauty in and out. As some advice, it is good to have an inspiration and motivation to conduct this particular healthy act of living. You can look for reasons like work, family, and love life and even friend and relationship concerns. It is a common fact that people will only accept you based on their first impression, and it is true that they cannot appreciate you as a person at a first glance. This is just a sample of motivation that you can use for you to immediately realize the importance of body image for the public's eyes.

Work habits need a lot of effort and energy execution. This reason can be used as a motivation for you to pursue living healthier while having a good body. As long as you exercise and eat appropriate types of food, you can generate positive system for your body such as intelligence and energy. As a result, you will no longer have to worry about the outcomes and accomplishments that will soon happen after you perform your job efficiently and effectively accompanied with a suitable amount of push and motivations.

Relationship will never have a good foundation if both partners do not possess the motivation to become a good person in relation to inside and outside appearance. It is better to be aware of how you can make yourself a good person and that it will also reflect on how you appear from the outside. Body image can also be one of the greatest motivations for a relationship to become stronger in terms of foundation. Yes love is more important, but maintaining a considerable appearance can generate more passion in love. As a matter of fact, body image can be more beneficial because it can make people that are in a relationship be in a more passionate state of romance when making love which is very healthy for love, connection, and communication.

Your family, especially your children, need your time and effort when the day ends after long and busy working hours. In this case, it is a motivation for you to become more energetic because your work is not the only entity that needs your full attention. It is better to patronize healthy living by means of exercising to promote the beneficial effects for your family that can only possibly delivered by a good image of body.

CHAPTER 5- CHOOSE A DIET PLAN TO EXTREME WEIGHT LOSS

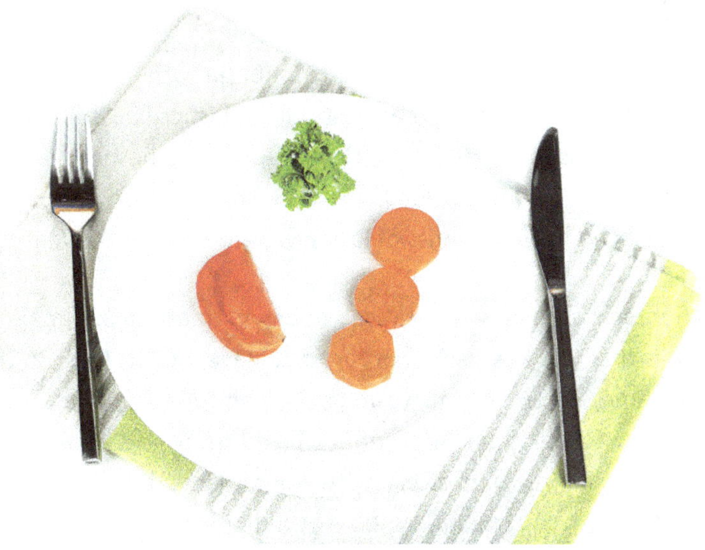

Sticking with your plans is beneficial when seriously depending on your target accomplishments. By living a healthy lifestyle, there is also a great chance of living a wealthy and comfortable way of life. So when the time comes that you decide to start working out with your Weight Loss Goals, you must never stop trying and practicing the system that can provide you opportunities for a lifetime. Gaining a lot of benefits is also possible by focusing your time and dedication towards making your weight satisfying, not only for the eye of other people, but also for the betterment of your health and life.

Tips to Stick with It

In maintaining a good focus on your plans of Weight Loss Goals, you must first right down all of your reasons, specific practices, and how and when you will be doing these diets and exercises. Writing these things down will give you an advantage, not letting you sway off track. In this way, you can also monitor the achievements that you have achieved every time you practice this healthy hobby of yours. Since you write down all your plans, you can also be more flexible in the case that you will be skipping some parts of it.

Realize your goal as a realistic one; in other words, make it attainable to the fact that you will not sacrifice too much. It is better to visualize things that can happen in the near future since anticipation will never lead you to depression. When you focus on these achievable benefits of losing weight you will prevent stress.

There are a lot of ways that can help you to attain and maintain the goals that you have set in order to achieve weight loss. But most of the time, in regards to your goals maintenance, these plans are difficult to perform. In accordance, there are additional acts that must be performed along with your plans. These practices can contribute to making your settled plans nice and safe. In accordance, these additives are proven to be effective in all conditions of the body structure.

Stick With Your Goals

Sleeping 7-8 hours is one of the healthy ways to stick with your plans. As long as you have complete hours of sleep, there is a great possibility that you can obtain energy that is sufficient for your target objectives. Another benefit that you can obtain when you have complete sleep is the focus that is needed by your mind to perform better work. As you practice this particular act, there is no way that you will fail on your plans. In accordance, you will never feel easily exhausted since you have the power that you need before and after working hours.

Another factor that can help you achieve your goals is the presence of people that will give you reasons to continue working out with your plans and goals. Make sure that they will not influence your activities that will make your plans invisible which is very inconsiderable. Bad influential people commonly offer activities that are unhealthy and can ruin your healthy lifestyle. Perfect partners for your achieving purposes are the ones that can share knowledge and practice with you.

You can promote these plans of yours to your friends and family. As long as you let them know your objectives in these healthy practices, there is no way that you cannot find a person that is interested and will come with you during each and every work-out session of yours. This factor can also help you avoid people that can easily influence and ruin your plans. Have some dinner with your friends and family, in this way, you can open up about your fitness plans, and who knows, maybe some of them already perform this healthy act which is very inviting to consider.

Eating enough food is beneficial for the reason that it will supply you with nutrients, vitamins, and minerals which are good for your energy, and mental and emotional concerns. In this way, you will never lose strength which can provide you with energy and prevent you from being totally exhausted. In addition, you will not feel starved after every work-out session that you attend. As you lose your fat, you can now replace it easily with nutrients that can supply you with nutrients.

Positive results are achievable and can be realized in no time, of course, when you are dedicated, focused on the procedures, and always looking forward for a better tomorrow and the beneficial results of being persistent. Although there are huge hindrances that might force you to stop trying, there are still numerous reasons and outcomes which will help you visualize things that can make you continue and maintain the good status of your plans. Together with these reasons, you will never have to feel some difficulty while being responsible for conducting your goals. As a result, you can now obtain the most positive result which you were targeting from the very first place.

The Benefits

Huge plans seem to be unachievable, but when you have the perseverance to do them, there is nothing impossible pertaining to the process that you have to overcome and practice almost every day. Although there are times which will make you feel exhausted and stressed in regards to your target objectives, as you think positive results, skills, knowledge and you capabilities will just boost the limit which is helpful in accomplishing the tasks that you have to do.

Vague goals are existent most of the time, especially when you are just starting the task. But never give up, along with the operation of your plans, in the process that makes you educated and aware, there is a great chance for you to make these goals visible and reachable. As a result, you can now make your objectives well-settled and written in your organizational diagram. This process will help you not to be confused in terms of your work-out days pertaining to the following program that you are following. This program is being planned by professional fitness trainers. Do not worry for they will help you be flexible in terms of schedule concerns.

Action plans will become more productive and effective as you continue working with your plan; this is a fact that is proven and a tested system which is being conducted by a lot of people who deals with the same objectives as you. Never stop struggling for your goal and you will never regret the result that will come up after every session. As you continue, little by little, you will notice that there will be changes in your lifestyle and the figure of your body.

Identifying consequences is not just a risk or problem that might force you to stop trying; it is also a beneficial factor that will push you more to go through. You will never know the result when you just foresee it; you have to try at least under a considerable amount of time. As you perform, you will never have guilt to yourself that you've never tried and practice and no longer achieve the real results of your plans.

Rewards are attainable and can always be realized as possible as you can. Hard work deserves some credit, so start living healthy, and in no time, you will be fulfilled with the results of happiness.

CHAPTER 6- EXTREME WEIGHT LOSS DOESN'T MEAN EXTREME STARVATION

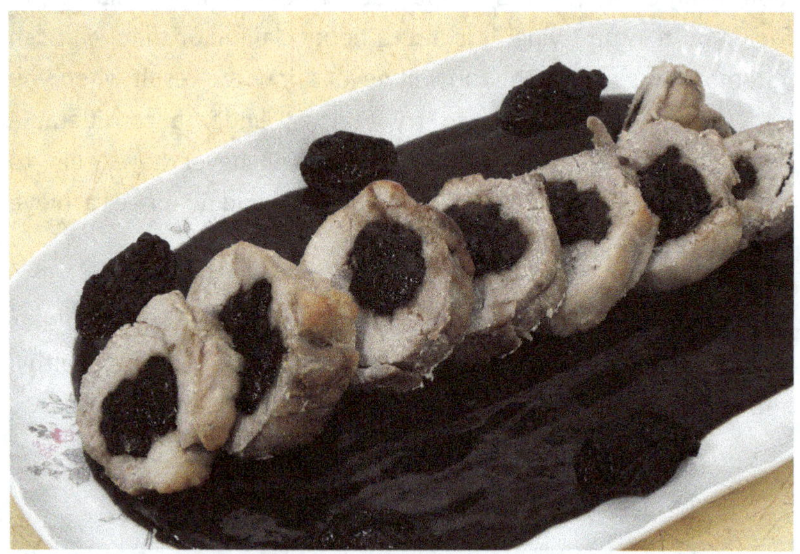

Trying to lose weight can be tough. Trying to lose weight fast can be even more of a challenge. If you think you have to starve yourself or endlessly exercise you'll be happy to learn that's not so.

Preparing for your weight loss program can make a huge difference in your success. When you take the time to evaluate your weight loss needs you'll be able to better chose the best diet and exercise program for you. Your metabolism is the key to your weight loss, which is why you need to discover how fast your metabolism is. There are plenty of free metabolism calculators you can use.

What many don't realize is that to enjoy the maximum weight loss two 15 minute cardio workouts 3 to 4 times a week, combined with some weight training or resistant training on 2 to 3 times a week will result in maximizing your weight loss. The best fast weight loss combines exercise with reduced calorie intake. It will provide you with the quickest results. As you build muscle, you'll it takes more calories to maintain that muscle and so you'll lose more fat.

Don't waste your time with crunches. All you'll do is develop muscle under the fat and you'll actually look fatter. Cardio workouts are ten times more effective so take advantage of them. There's no need to have to spend any money to enjoy your cardiac workout other than a pair of comfortable shoes. Walking briskly is an excellent cardio workout. Of course, you can add cycling, jogging, running, or other activities, which you enjoy.

The best diet is a healthy diet. That means avoiding processed foods and eating plenty of fresh fruits and vegetables, as well as quality protein (poultry and fish) and complex carbs. Then all you need to do is take in fewer calories than you use.

You can do this by either eating less or by exercising more. There's really no big secret here. If you reduce your calorie intake start with a 100 to 200 calorie reduction. Never drop more than 500 calories or you risk scaring your body into starvation mode. When that happens, you'll not lose a pound.

To learn you can lose weight quickly is rather exciting. It's great to discover it doesn't have to take months to lose those pounds. In fact, you can easily lose 3 to 5 pounds a week and you can do it without any risk to your health. In no time, at all you'll be leaner, thinner, and more toned.

What the Experts Say about Losing Weight Fast

Weight gain is frustrating when you're trying everything you can think of to shed those pounds. You watch what you eat, you exercise, and still...the pounds stay. Everyone knows that eating too much, eating fried or fatty foods, eating sugary foods, drinking alcohol and soda can lead to excess weight gain, but even those who avoid all these things find themselves putting on the pounds.

So how can you lose weight fast in a healthy manner? The good news is it isn't as difficult as you might have thought. According to some experts, a few key techniques can help you quickly shed those extra pounds. Losing weight quickly requires more than eating less and exercising more. To lose weight fast you need to combine exercise, diet, dietary supplements, and emotional support. Here are a few more techniques to help you lose weight:

* Listen to your body – Adjust your exercise and your diet to correspond with your goals and your body.

* Set goals that are realistic – Make sure you set goals that can be achieved; stay motivated, and stay focused.

* Drink more water – Drinking water removes toxins from the body. It also keeps you feeling full.

* Eat more fiber – Fiber help to fill you faster and you stay feeling full for longer.

* Remain consistent – Your success depends on remaining consistent with your plan.

* Stay away from packaged and processed foods – these foods have little nutrition, too much fat, too much sodium, and they are just plain bad for you and your waistline.

There are all kinds of diet supplements on the market. Some may be helpful, some are of no value, and some are dangerous. Before you take any diet supplements make sure you do your homework and understand how and if they can help. Quick weight loss can occur without the use of supplements.

If you've ever watched "The Biggest Loser," you'll know that you can safely lose significant weight in one month if you want to. It's important to realize that losing weight involves more than just losing fat. Weight loss involves the body's water, muscle tissue, and bone mass.

Rapid weight loss can entail dehydration, loose skin, cramping, diarrhea, and fatigue. So while you can safely lose weight quickly, you can only do this providing you understand your nutritional needs vs. your weight loss, and what your limits are. You should also never undertake a weight loss program without first discussing it with your physician.

How to Quickly Get Lean

You'll be happy to know that there's no reason you can't build muscle and lose fat fast. Once you've turned fat into muscle, with a few changes to lifestyle you can look lean and fit for the rest of your life. But how does one get started in building muscle and losing fat? Glad you asked! And there's great news because you can do it quickly.

The quickest way to build your muscle mass is to get stronger. Any type of strength training will work. There's weight training that involves dumbbells, barbells, and exercises like squats. You can use either free weights or weight machines.

As you build muscle, your body fat will decrease. Along with strength training, you need 30 minutes of cardio exercise three times a week. The goal here is not to exhaust yourself but rather to burn fat. When doing your cardio you should be breathing heavier than you normally would but you should not be gasping for air. You should always talk to your doctor before starting any exercise program.

You can't build your muscles unless you are feeding them properly, and when you are eating right, you'll also be losing fat. Your nutrition needs to include at least 1 gram of protein per pound of body weight daily. So things like poultry, fish, and eggs are good sources of protein. You also need the good fats, which include omega 3, 6, and 9 found in things like olive oil and fish oil. Make sure you are eating plenty of veggies, especially the greens. Steam doesn't cook. All kinds of fruit are good for you, and you'll also want to make sure your eating only whole grain foods. Water is critical to your fast fat loss program. Stay away from packaged foods and fast foods, and get rid of the soda.

As well as eating healthy, you are going to have to reduce your calorie intake. Don't do anything drastic because that triggers the body to think it's in starvation mode and it actually becomes more difficult to lose those pounds. Instead, reduce gradually. The first week cut out 500kcal.

After a week check to see if you've lost weight and reduce more as necessary. Never cut more calories if you see you are losing weight.

Keeping a journal can help to motivate you and stay on track. There are even free websites that allow you to track your progress online. Loosing

The Secret to Lose Weight and Build Muscle Fast

Weight loss – there's a lot of buzz around it, but how do you lose weight and build muscle fast? Glad you asked! It's time the secret was out.

The weight loss industry is a multibillion dollar industry and they'd like everyone to believe there's some big secret that they know and you don't. That' how they sell you the magic weight loss formulas. It's time you knew the truth about what it takes to lose weight and build muscle fast.

Muscle vs. Fat

If you are trying to lose weight and build muscle and you want to do it fast, crash diets that seriously restrict your caloric intake aren't what you need. When you lose weight while dieting, you lose muscle and fat. Exercise will preserve your muscle and build new muscle. You need to eat healthy and incorporate a vigorous exercise regime into your daily life. That will build muscle and you can watch the fat shrink away.

The Right Foods to Build Your Muscles

If you want to build your muscles, you are going to have to feed them, and not just any food – the right foods. Proteins are key to building your muscles. This is why bodybuilders use protein shakes to bulk up. But don't ignore carbs, because they are also important to building muscles. The key to losing weight and building muscles quickly is to eat a balanced diet. You should be taking in two grams of protein per kilogram of body weight if you are following a serious exercise regime, however if you are not exercising you should be taking in no more than .8 grams per kilogram of body weight.

Calorie Counting

Without ever cutting calories, increasing your exercise and you can see an amazing reduction in weight loss. The formula to weight loss is really no secret. You must use more calories than you take in. So start paying attention and make sure you are burning up more than you are taking in. You also need to make better food choices – healthier choices mean you'll have more energy and feel fuller.

Building Muscle

You aren't going to bulk up overnight. If that's your goal and you put the time in you'll see the result in a few weeks, without any magic potions or pills. Start slow, with weights you are comfortable working with. Always do your exercises properly. Match your goals and your training to get the results you expect.

There you have it. There's really no big secret. The right mix of diet and exercise and you'll be toned and lighter in no time at all. You really can lose weight and build muscle fast.

Which Diets Are Best to Lose Weight Fast?

For most of us those pounds go on faster than they come off. But which diets are best to lose weight fast? Glad you asked! When it comes to fast weight loss some diets work better than others, and regardless of your diet choice it's important to add an exercise component too.

It's also important to choose a diet that you can stick to. There's no point in choosing a diet considered a fast weight loss program if you can't stand the foods that are in it.

Let's look at some of your diet options others have found useful to lose weight fast:

Scarsdale Diet – This is a diet known for its choices, which makes it easier to stick to. It's also a good choice if you're the type of person that doesn't want to be going around hungry. There's no weighting, counting, or measuring. Just follow the simple menus.

The Lemonade Diet – If you're a person with a strong willpower you might consider this combination cleanse diet.

The Cabbage Soup Diet – This is a popular choice for anyone who doesn't want to be on a diet for more than seven days. It's cheap and it's repetitive. It works but you had better like cabbage.

The Three Day Diet – This is a great way to lose 10 pounds in three days.

What one has to remember is that these while these diets have worked well for many who want to lose weight fast, they don't necessarily lead to long term weight loss if they aren't combined with healthy lifestyle choice? That includes nutritious eating and exercise.

Your exercise program doesn't have to be costly or difficult. A brisk walk that gets your heart rate up and some weight training right in your living room will do the trick. Resistance exercises are great for toning muscles, as are squats, pushups, and lunges. You might want to add a set of dumbbells to the mix but you can also used cans. Be creative. Of course, for some the gym membership is a way to keep them focused and on track. Whatever works for you. That's what's important.

Extreme Weight Loss Made Easy With Simple Steps
While diets may start to see the pounds melt away fast, you need to make healthy food choices to enjoy the long term benefits. That includes eating fresh veggies and fruits, good protein such as poultry and fish, and avoiding packaged and processed foods.

With just a little effort you can look and feel better in no time at all. Watch those pounds melt away.

CHAPTER 7- MOTIVATION TO EXTREME WEIGHT LOSS

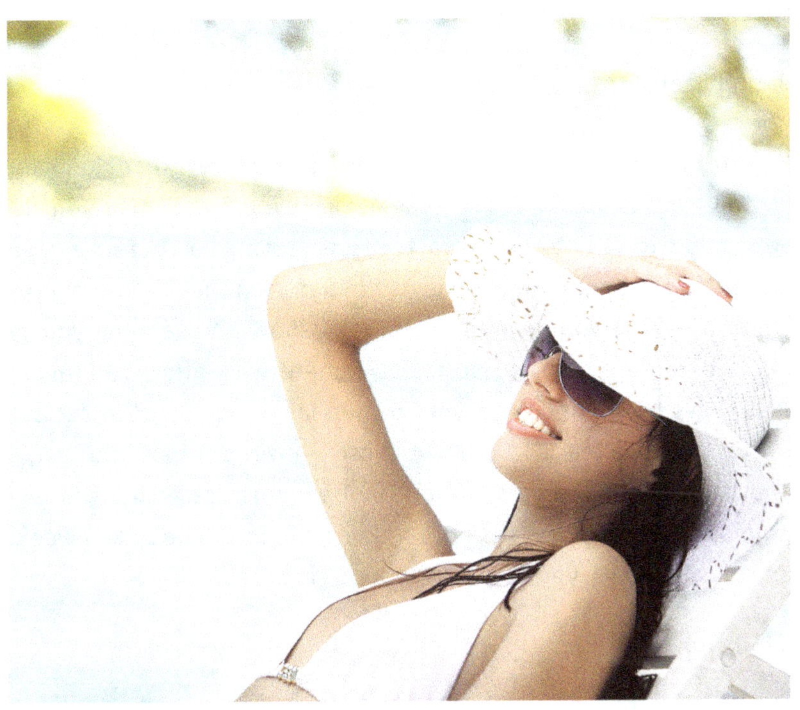

If you find yourself needing to lose weight, you're not alone. But saying you want to lose weight and actually watching those pounds disappear are two different things. Let's be honest – we're creatures of habit and we don't make change easy. That's why you want to use these 10 ways to motivate yourself to lose weight fast.

1. Play the If I Do vs. the If I Don't Game

Grab a piece of paper. Draw a line down the middle and one side write "If I Do" and on the other side write, "If I don't." You're looking into the future now. What will your life be like a month, a year, five years from now. If you take action and lose the weight or if you don't take action and lose the weight. Be honest with yourself.

For example, if I do lose the weight in one year I'll be able to eat what I want without worrying about getting fat. Or If I don't lose the weight in five years, I'm likely to be diabetic. This is a great exercise for motivating yourself – just be real!

2. Don't Let Anything Get in Your Way

If you have decided to lose the weight and look great don't let anything get in your way. You can achieve your goal when you set your mind to it but you need to have a plan. For example, you decide you are going to exercise 30 minutes on the stationary bike while watching your favorite television show. Or perhaps you've decided you are going to go f a 15 minute walk after work every day. Don't let excuses stop you from doing what you have set out to do. It's really easy to say put it off. I'm tired, I have company, and I have to do laundry. Stick to your guns and you'll see the pounds start to roll off. It's not unrealistic to lose 5 pounds a week. So in just a month you can be 20 pounds lighter.

3. Reward Yourself

If any of you have ever trained a dog you know how important rewards are. They're important to you too so be sure to set some. For example, if I lose 20 pounds in two months I will treat myself to a meal at my favorite restaurant.

4. Bet With Yourself

The more extreme you make the bet, the more you have to lose. Go t a friend and tell them, "If I don't lose 20 pounds in the next two months I'll walk your dog for a month." If you want to motivate yourself even more "Go to your boss and tell him if you don't lose 20 pounds in the next two months you'll work for free for two weeks.

There are four great ways to motivate yourself to get the job done. You can lose that extra weight and you can do it fast.

The Best 3 Tips to Build Muscle and Lose Body Fat

If you want to build muscle and lose body fat these three tips can accomplish both. After all, you want to lose weight (body fat) without sacrificing muscle. Good news – this can be done you properly tackle the challenge. However, to gain muscle while losing weight you really have to have your nutrition and exercise program right on the money.

You also have to understand that muscle weights more than fat. Therefore, as you build more muscle your weight may actually go up while you find your waist size going down. In the last decade, there have been significant advancements in the nutritional advances, which is why today's bodybuilder can stay lean and muscular twelve months of the year. It's all about your calorie intake vs. your calorie burn.

It's about balance. You need to take in enough calories to lose weight and gain muscle but not so many calories that you gain fat. You also need to find the right workout balance. Go for a lower number of sets and reps using a heavier weight. You should train each muscle group only one every week. On top of weight training your cardio workout is important. It needs to be intense and short.

The best 3 tips to build muscle and lose body fat are:

1. Figure out how many calories you use a day and then make sure you are not taking in more calories than that.

2. Ensure your weight training is heavy so that it will stimulate muscle growth. If you don't use heavy weights you won't stimulate

the growth you desire. Weight training can be accomplished with a set of free weights. Dumbbells can be purchased cheap, and you can even get creative and use cans. Squats, lunges, and sit-ups are a good weight training exercises that cost you nothing.

3. Make sure your cardio workout is short and intense. It's a common misconception that the longer cardio sessions do a better job of burning fat and preserving the lean muscle mass.

Losing weight and developing muscles can be done quickly and efficiently without jeopardizing your health. While there are all kinds of supplements on the market promoting fast weight loss. Far too many of these supplements are all hype and no substance. Many others are little more than vitamins. Before you spend your money, it pays to do your homework.

From Fat to Fit What You Need to Know

Have you discovered the secret to quick weight loss? The truth is there is no secret. What there is are many unique ways that share similar characteristics. It's time you learned what you need to know to go from fat to fit.

Deciding on a weight loss, muscle building program has a lot to do with your personal preferences and tastes. It should also be based on your level of commitment. After all, there's no point in choosing a program that requires you to work out every day when you are only willing to work out three times a week.

There are all kinds of fad diets on the market that would like you to believe they have something that no one else has. The reality is most of these diets are similar. And while they have worked for many the key is being able to keep the weight off long term. If you decide to use a fad diet then you also need to have a long term plan in place and you need to be ready to make the lifestyle changes necessary to keep the weight off.

The truth is if you are looking to lose weight and gain muscle mass quickly, there are only a few tried and true way to do this. Here are some great tips to help you burn fat and build muscle.

1. Four days a week, you need to do 45 minutes of moderate free weight strength training.

2. Add high intensity cardio workouts that are 15 minutes in length and done three days a week.

3. Incorporate a nutritious well balanced diet into your life. Avoid junk food, processed food, and convenience food which has little nutritional value and far too many wasted calories.

4. You should not eat two hours before bedtime. Eating too late turns these calories into fat.

5. Drink lots of water. In fact, you should be drinking a gallon a day. Water removes the toxins from your body and it also fills you up. Have a glass of water before you sit down to eat and you'll eat far less. Got the munchies, drink a glass of water. Water also provides the necessary hydration to your muscles.

Building muscles and losing fat is not a onetime occurrence. It requires you to make some changes to your lifestyle. To keep the weight off you will need to continue to exercise and eat healthy. The good news is losing the weight isn't nearly as difficult as many would have you believe. Why not start today?

How Cardio Training Can Lose Weight and Build Muscle Quickly

The topic of losing weight can often elicit "groans." There's no need you know. In fact, did you know that cardio training can lead to quickly building muscle mass and losing weight. Cardio training can be as simple or as complex as you like. Walking, jogging, and cycling are all goof forms of aerobic exercise that can quickly burn body fat. Aerobic exercises are a great choice for the entire body.

There's all kinds of sites promoting the "secret to successful weight loss" online but it's really not as complicated as we might want to make it out to be. If you want to lose weight quickly then you must change the ration between calorie intake and calorie use. You can either increase your exercise or decrease your calories. The best plan of attack is to combine the two. Reduce your calories by no more than 500 and increase your activity with a daily 30 minutes of cardio a day.

When you build muscle you burn fat. Strength training builds muscle. Squats, lunges, and pushups require no equipment is very effective. Free weights are also very effective – dumbbells can be purchased for cheap and cans always work too. Don't make this more expensive or complicated than it has to be.

Fat burning aerobic exercise is different than recreational exercise. For example Tennis and golf are recreational exercise and won't do a thing for your weight loss, or very little. Then again aerobic exercise such as running, walking, and jogging for 30 minutes without stopping will get the heart pumping and the fat melting.

For awhile it was thought that low intensity exercises would do the job of burning fat but that myth was quickly dismissed. If you don't get your heart rate up you won't burn fat. When you have a high intensity aerobic workout you will consume around 70% of the body's energy. This means calories are burnt and that includes fat cells.

Your cardio workout can be as little as 10 to 15 minutes but a 45 to 60 minute workout is the most effective for burning fat. Don't think for a minute that more is better, because after 60 minutes the amount of weight loss actually goes down not up.

Cardio training can lose weight and build muscles quickly but when it comes to healthy weight loss that you can maintain you'll want to ensure you have a healthy lifestyle.

The Best Way to Enjoy Quick Weight Loss

Weight loss is a battle many of us find ourselves facing. Whether its 10 pounds or 100 pounds you can do, and you can enjoy quick weight loss too. Let's look at some great ways to speed up your weight loss.

One way to speed up your weight loss is to speed up your metabolism. One sure fire way to increase your metabolism is to get active. When you increase your muscle mass you speed up your metabolism. Another way to boost your metabolism is eat small amounts more often.

Rather than three meals a day, go for six small meals a day. Eating foods that are high in protein and foods that are spicy can both improve your metabolism. Give up coffee and start drinking green tea. There are all kinds of evidence that green tea speeds up the metabolism. You should set an alarm to go off every four hours to remind you to eat. Sound ridiculous? Well it's not. This technique ensures you eat smaller meals throughout the day, an effective metabolism booster.

Finally have a sauna. Being hot can boost the metabolism by 20%. You should always talk to your physician before using a sauna. A very hot bath can help too. While it may not be as effective as a sauna, it still helps.

Losing weight is all about change. You need to change your eating habits, your exercise patterns, and your lifestyle choices. You need to create a plan of action, motivate yourself, and then get going. Throw your body a curve ball and change things up rather than always doing the same thing. With this method you'll see the fastest weight loss. And remember to make positive choices in your life now that you'll be able to do for the rest of your life.

Here's a little secret many don't know about. Lemon juice speeds up weight loss. It contains citric acid, which slows gastric emptying time so you feel full longer, and eat less. Your diet should be high in protein, complex carbs, and fiber, while it should be low in fat and simple carbs. Most of us have trigger foods we just can't put down once we start eating them. Storing these foods in the freezer makes it harder to carry out that behavior thereby breaking the cycle. Finally, you need to incorporate exercise into your weight loss program. Cardio exercises combined with weight training will optimize and tone your muscles while burning the unwanted fat. You can easily lose 3 to 5 pounds a week and those numbers can be much higher if you are truly committed.

From Fat to Slim In 5 Easy Steps

Weight loss programs always seem to generate controversy and this one is likely no different. If you're like most of us you don't really care about the science, you just want to lose the pounds. Let's look at how you can go from fat to slim in 5 easy steps and with only 10 to 15 minutes a day

1. Start Slow – You may be surprised to learn this is one of the most important things you can do because if your enthusiasm gets the better of you, you'll find yourself burnt out. It's easier to add more exercise than it is to take away.

2. Choosing the Type of Cardio Exercise – You'll be much more successful if you choose exercise that you enjoy or at least think you'll enjoy. For example, if you never liked riding bike in the past, taking up cycling is likely a bad choice with a short outcome. You have many options. You can join a gym and circuit train or strength strain, but you can also lose those pounds without spending a dime. Walk...walk...walk some more – get your heart rate up but not so much that you can't hold a conversation.

3. Add Some Strength Exercises - Add a little strength training at home using cans or anything else you can find with a bit of weight. And of course, for just a few bucks you can buy dumbbells. Crunches, pushups, and squats require no equipment whatsoever and they are very good at toning and slimming. While they may sound too simple to be effective, that's not the case. They work fast and they work well.

4. Exercise Every Day – You hear all kinds of instructions about when and how you should exercise. The bottom line is just do it. The shorter the period of time the more likely you are to do it but the more often you'll need to do it. So if you are going to work out for 10 to 15 minutes a day you need to do it every day to be successful.

5. Just get moving – Don't plan, don't spend weeks trying to figure out the best plan of action, just put on your shoes and get out there and go for a walk or start doing jumping jacks in the middle of your living room. Just get moving, because when you are moving

you are building muscle and when you are toning and building muscle you are burning fat.

There you have it – from fat to slim in 5 easy steps. Now that you know how to lose weight and build muscle fast, so get busy.

CHAPTER 8- GAIN MUSCLE, LOSE WEIGHT

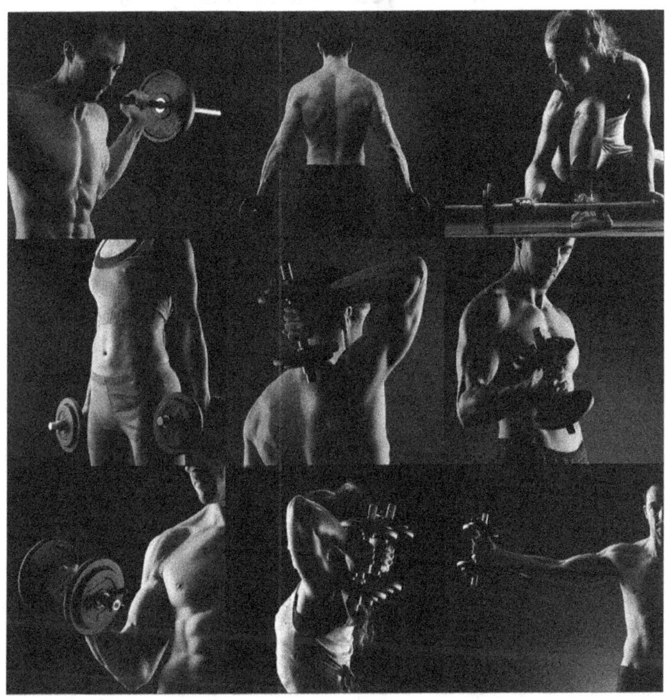

So you've decided it's time to lose those extra pounds – good for you! We thought It was time to share the down and dirty on how to gain muscle while losing fat fast! These simple steps will have you leaner in no time at all.

1. Drink Away

Don't get too excited. We're not talking about beer, but rather water. If you've never really understood the importance of this clear, tasteless liquid it's time you did. Every process in the body used water. You should drink at least a gallon a day. Take a bottle with you wherever you go. It detoxifies the body so that your organs run optimally and it fills you so you'll eat less.

2. Be a Goal Setter

Until you actually set goals about how much body fat you wish to lose and how much muscle you want to gain, you'll never actually take the first step needed to achieve your goal. Instead you'll spend your days dreaming about what your body would look like and what life would be like if you were leaner, more muscular, and more toned. Set your goal and then put a plan into action and you'll be successful.

3. Eat Small Meals

Rather than 3 large meals a day, you should eat 5 to 6 small meals consisting of moderate carbs, low fat, and high protein. This will keep your metabolism optimized and calories burning more efficiently. You should eat 50% of your calories from protein, 40% from carbs, and 10% from fats.

4. Turn Your 30 Minute Cardio Workout Into Two 15 Minute Workouts 4 Times a Week

Rather than doing a 30 minute cardio workout do two 15 minute cardio workouts. It's easier to have an intense 15 minute cardio workout twice a day than a 30 minute session. Warm up for a couple of minutes and cool down for a couple of minutes leaving you with about 11 minutes of workout. You should only do cardio on the days you aren't doing weight training.

5. Do Weight Training 3 Times a Week

6. Weight training builds muscle. Weight training doesn't burn fat, but muscles will burn more calories to maintain the muscles. If you want to lose fat, simply make your weight training or resistance training a priority.

7. Calculate Your Calorie Needs

To lose body fat calculate your calorie needs. Then reduce your calorie intake or increase your calorie output. A good starting point is around 200 calories and never more than 500 calories or your body will go into starvation mode and store fat.

These six tips are a great way to gain muscle while losing fat fast.

Build Muscle Lose Fat Fast and Feel Great

Whether this is the first time you've decided to lose weight or your hundredth attempt you can do this. You can build muscle, lose fat fast, and feel great. So how do you go about doing this? Glad you asked!

It all begins with building muscle. Now don't worry you're not going to turn yourself into the incredible hulk. Women in particular worry that they'll become too muscular and that just doesn't happen without some very specialized work.

As you build muscle, your weight may actually increase. Don't worry; this is okay, because muscle actually weighs more than fat. As your muscles develop, your body will begin to burn fat faster. Your weight training is really quite simple – squats, pushups, and free weights are all the equipment you need.

You're going to that weight training with cardio exercises to burn fat. Either 30 minutes a day or two 15 minute sessions will be enough cardio to enjoy the benefits. Cardio is as simple as a brisk walk. Of course, there are all kinds of cardio exercises including jogging, cycling, circuit training, and tons of other excellent aerobic exercises. A treadmill can be a great investment because of the convenience of that walk indoors no matter what the weather.

Your cardio should raise your heart rate but not make you out of breath.

You will also need to look at your diet. To build muscle you need to make sure you are taking 25% to 30% of your calories in protein. You'll want to avoid fats, and add plenty of fiber to your diet. Fiber is filling and so you'll eat less. Avoid eating all processed and packaged foods, which contain little nutrition. Instead, stick to fresh fruits and vegetables, poultry, fish, and lean meat cuts.

For many of us, belly fat is our biggest enemy. It's also the hardest to lose. Don't make the mistake of thinking that as long as you do hundreds of crunches will do the job. All that will happen is the muscle under the fat will develop and your belly will look larger. Cardio exercises are needed to burn belly fat!

Great, we've covered how to build muscle and lose fat fast, but there's more to it than exercise and caloric intake. One of the biggest reasons why weight loss fails is failing to have a plan, so get your plan in place. Finally, don't wait to get motivated. Set goals, reward yourself, get up, and get moving. Before you know it, you'll have shed those extra pounds.

How to Lose Weight Fast and Easy

If you've heard it once you've heard it a dozen times – fad diets don't result in permanent weight loss. But what about when you want to lose a few pounds fast. It's hard not to try the Cabbage Soup Diet or Lose 21 Pounds in 21 Days Diet. While these diets might work is this really safe weight loss and will it last? According to NBC's Biggest Loser medical doctor Dr. Michael Dansinger, there's nothing wrong with rapid weight loss.

Losing 20 pounds in a week because of an aggressive exercise and easting program that involves hours a day of exercise combined with healthy eating choices and restricted calorie intake can result in exactly this kind of weight loss. However, such a program should never be undertaken without first getting your physicians approval.

Even without taking it to the extreme losing 3 to 5 pounds a week can easily be accomplished. Losing weight fast is really as simple as a math formula. You must burn more calories than you take in. A deficit of 500 calories seems to be the recommended and can be accomplished by reducing your calorie intake and increasing your physical activity.

If you want to lose those pounds faster than exercise more and eat less. Around 1100 calories combined with one hour of exercise a day will lead to a loss of 3 to 5 pounds in the first week. If you weigh more than 250 pounds then the amount will be more. Great news – According to Dr. Michael Dansinger, the more fat you have to lose the faster it will come off.

Did you know you can lose up to 5 pounds in fluid just by reducing starch and sodium intake. While cutting back calories has the greatest effect on weight loss it's important to not do any drastic reduction or you'll put your body into starvation mode and you'll lose nothing. Dieticians recommend not going below 1,200 calories a day.

5 Tips to Quick and Effective Weight Loss:

1. Drink plenty of water. You can reduce hunger by drinking more water.

2. Eat plenty of low calorie fruits and vegetables. They'll make you feel full.

3. Eat six small meals a day rather than three large ones.

4. Get rid of all those foods that are bad for your waist (and your health) by removing them from the house.

5. Weigh yourself daily and track the food you take in – it will keep you focused on your weight loss.

Now that you know how to lose weight fast and easy, what are you waiting for?

Did You Know You Can You Lose Fat and Gain Muscle at the Same Time

It's a common question – Can you lose fat and gain muscle at the same time. Great news, the answer is emphatically "yes." When you build muscle and tone up your body will use the fat to feed those muscles so overall, it's a win-win for you.

You can't gain muscle and lose fat at the same time, but you can do both at the same time. Let me explain. To lose fat you need to do cardio exercises, eat a low fat, low carb, and low calorie diet, and do weight training or resistance training. To gain muscle you should do very little cardio exercise, eat a high car, high protein, high calorie diet, and do weight training. As you can see, they are complete opposites, which is why trying to gain muscle and lose fat at the same time simply doesn't work.

The secret is to implement phases. There's the muscle building phase, and then there is the fat losing phase. Don't worry if you see your weight increasing. Muscle weighs more than fat and so you can find yourself weighing more and yet losing inches around the waist.

When you are in the muscle building phase you will be eating more calories and your diet will include high proteins, complex carbs, and good fats. Many women worry they will become too muscular. The odds of that happening are very slim, but what you will do is develop strength and tone your body.

When you are in the fat training phase, you'll be reducing your calories, eating lower carbs, but still eating protein and good fats. So you see protein and good fats remains constant. As you move into the fat training phase, you're now only worried about maintaining the strength you've developed. Your focus now is to melt away the fat and because you've been building muscle the fat is now much easier to melt away.

Your fat phase involves cardio exercises. Did you know a brisk walk is considered a cardio exercise? It's simple, it has no costs associated with it, and it's effective. Cycling, jogging, and running are other good cardio exercises. Basically, any exercise that gets your heart rate up is a good cardio exercise. Remember, you should not be out of breath when doing your cardio exercises.

So you see you can lose fat and gain muscle at the same time. It all begins by putting your plan into action and then getting motivated. So what are you waiting for?

10 Super Foods to Help You Quickly Build Muscle and Lose Weight

In order to build muscle and lose weight you need a variety of veggies, carbs, fruits, proteins, and healthy fats. In order to quickly build muscle and lose weight you need 10 super foods.

1. Whole Eggs – Eggs are one of the cheapest super foods offering you an excellent source of protein. The cholesterol that we hear so

much about isn't a problem. If you have cholesterol problems lower your body fat not the eggs you consume.

2. Flax Seeds – Here's an excellent source of fiber, omega 3, and protein. Grind the flax seeds and sprinkle on your berries or yogurt. Don't use flax oil as it's unstable and has no fiber benefits.

3. Quinoa – In South America Quinoa is considered the king of grains. The fiber and protein in Quinoa is higher than that in oats and rice, plus its gluten free.

4. Mixed Nuts – Nuts are packed with mono and polyunsaturated fats, fiber, proteins, Vitamin e, potassium, zinc, and magnesium. Nuts are dense in calories so if you are skinny and looking to put on a few pounds these will do it.

5. Wild Salmon – Omega 3 fatty acids are found in salmon, as well as providing 20 grams of protein per 100 gram serving.

6. Fish Oil – Taking fish oil can reduce inflammation in the body, increase testosterone levels, and lower body fat. Take 900mg per day. It's hard to get this level eating fish.

7. Berries – Fresh berries are a powerful antioxidant keeping you healthy and helping you to improve your weight loss.

8. Green Tea – Another strong antioxidant and a powerful natural diuretic. It can speed up fat loss, improve blood sugar, and prevent cancer.

9. Water – Something as simple water is considered a super food and vital to your weight loss program, muscle development, and health. You should drink at least 8 glasses a day.

10. Tomatoes – High in lycopene they are an excellent cancer preventer and a benefit in your strength training. You can't eat too many tomatoes!

These 10 super foods combined with an overall healthy diet, a cardiac workout, and some strength training and in no time you'll be pounds lighter. Super foods can help you to quickly build muscles and lose weight. Being overweight is hazardous to your health and to your self- esteem. Why not set your goals and get motivated? You'll be feeling better about your weight in no time at all.

5 Tips to Fast Weight Loss

Weight loss is a touchy subject for many of us. After all, it's a bit frustrating to see those pounds go on a lot easier than they come off and with so many different claims of fast weight loss it's hard to decipher what works and what doesn't. Check out these 5 tips to fast weight loss.

1. Make a Plan – Saying I want to lose weight isn't a plan for losing weight. Telling yourself you'll eat healthy starting tomorrow, or you'll start jogging next Monday, isn't a plan for action, and it's not going to help you lose those extra pounds. In fact, the failure rate is almost 100% when there is no plan. What's a plan look like? Well it goes something like this: I'm going to lose 10 pound in 35 days and I'm going to exercise for 30 minutes every day at 4:30pm.

2. Acai Berry – The buzz of Acai Berry seems to have traveled quickly around the globe. This is one of the best antioxidant foods out there and the Acai Berry Select Weight Loss Supplement has been talked about by Dr. Oz as being a successful tool by many.

3. Chew it Properly – If you're wondering what chewing has to be with weight loss you'll be surprised to learn that chewing your food 10 times before you swallow allows your body to better use the nutrient and it also means better digestion of foods leading to weight loss.

4. Drink Plenty of Water – When you drink adequate water your body is able to flush away harmful toxin. Water has no calories and the more of it you drink the fuller you'll feel. There are no calories in water. Drinking a large glass before you eat means you'll eat far less. And when you find yourself reaching for an unhealthy snack drink a glass or two of water and watch the urge disappear.

5. Resistance Training – With resistance training you muscles responds to the resistance placed on them. If you life weights there's tiny tears in the muscles which require energy to rebuild and that energy comes from the fat stored in your body. To lose weight you need to create a calorie deficit so when muscles use calories you lose pounds. It's not nearly as complicated as some might want to make it.

Fast weight loss isn't as difficult to accomplish as you might think. Put these 5 great tips to work and you'll see your waist start to shrink in no time.

10 Top Tips to Help You Quickly Lose Weight

Losing weight can be a real challenge. Doing it quickly and in a manner that's healthy is important, but not as difficult as you might think. Follow these 10 top tips to lose weight quickly.

1. Watch What you Eat – You should be keeping an eye on everything you put in your mouth. It's the garnishes, and the extras that can be packed with calories.

2. Burn off Those Extra Calories – To lose weight you need to take in fewer calories than you burn. As you track your calories if you are taking in more than you are burning you'll need to ramp up the exercise. This is important so don't let it out of your sight.

3. Fried Foods are Bad – If you want to lose weight fast, you need to avoid fried foods completely. Even if you drain or soak off the oil, it's within the food. To lose weight quickly take fried food out of your diet.

4. Don't Skip Meals – This is one of the worst things you can do while trying to lose weight quickly. If you skip meals, you will actually gain weight. Eat a minimum of four to six meals a day.

5. Only Fresh Fruit Juice – We all know how important it is to drink plenty of water but sometimes we have a craving for something other than water. In that case, you should choose fresh fruit juice that contains no added sweeteners, which translate to calories.

6. Increase Your Fiber – Fiber is really good for you and it is important in your weight loss program so make sure you are getting enough.

7. Go Vegetable Crazy – When it comes to weight loss vegetables are your best choice. While all veggies are good for you, leafy greens are your best choice. Make sure you include them in your salad. Fresh veggies contain the nutrients you need and they offer important fiber to the diet. They make great snack foods and can quickly take care of hunger pangs.

8. No Between Meal Snacks – Do not fall into the habit of snacks between meals. This is a common problem for people on the move. They get hungry and grab whatever junk food is nearest to take away the hunger pains. These are not only calories you don't need

or want; there is also a great deal of fat in these snack foods. Just eliminating junk food snacks and soda can easily lead to a 2 to 3 pound reduction a month, without doing anything else.

9. Your Diet Should Be Made Up of 30% Protein – If you are going to build muscle, you need protein. Muscle burns fat and so you've got a winning situation here.

10. Eat Smart – The difference between eating smart and eating to eliminate the feeling of hunger is the difference. Don't just eat to eat. Ask yourself if what you are about to eat is going to offer your body nutrition.

These 10 top tips will help you lose weight quickly. Losing weight doesn't have to be hard.

Build The Perfect Male Physique - Gain Muscle Lose Fat Quickly

How would you like to build the perfect male physique? Would you like to gain muscle and lose fat quickly? Then you've come to the right place. If you want to develop bigger muscles and get more ripped. If you want to develop a six pack or if you want to get rid of that extra fat you need two things from your body. Sound confusing? It's really not.

If you want to lose a lot of fat and gain a lot of muscle all at once it can be difficult. That's because they are at opposite ends of the scale. If you want to build new muscle your body will require additional energy, which means more food and more calories. To lose fat you need to eat less and that means fewer calories. So how can you do both.

In the early stages of building muscle and losing fat there's a bit of a balancing act. It starts by eating right. You will need to increase your calories to develop muscles. Increase your protein and decrease the fat in your diet. To maintain that muscle will take more energy and that means fat will be burned. In addition if you've lowered your caloric intake you'll see even quicker results.

What many don't know is that the more muscular you become the harder it gets to lose fat. But don't despair. It's all in the balance. On average men will gain approx. 9 pounds of muscle for every 16 pounds of fat. In the earliest stages you'll lose fat and gain muscle quicker. As you reach your body's upper limits your success will begin to decline.

If you've been fit before it will be much easier to lose fat and build muscles. Muscles have a memory and even if you've let them get out of shape they'll quickly fall back to their muscle memory if you decide to get back in shape. This is great news!

To gain muscle and lose fat quickly spend the first 5 weeks building muscle and then the next 3 or so weeks losing fat. There are two methods that work well for achieving your goals.

The Bracketing Method – You cycle your calorie intake and carb intake through the week depending on the kind of training you are doing.

The Sawtooth Method – This method involves losing fat and gaining muscle until you reach a body fat percentage you previously determined.

By the end of the 8 week period you'll be leaner, have less body fat, and look fantastic!

The truth is we can build muscle and lose weight fast. Failure often comes on the hands of poor information. There are 5 common myths about fast weight loss that you shouldn't believe.

Myth #1 – I overeat so there's no way I'll ever lose fat quickly.

Overeating is mostly the result of stress – when a person is worried, depressed, scared, sad, or anxious overeating is often the result. Decrease your stress and you'll be surprised at how fast you lose pound. Becoming physically active can lead to a loss in weight.

Myth #2 – My genetics mean I'll always be overweight.

Being fat isn't a result of your genetics. Yes some families may have a pattern of being overweight but you can overcome your genes and lose fat quickly. Your genetics don't control your weight, your lifestyle choices do. Watch a couple of episodes of "The Biggest Loser" if you want proof.

Myth #3 – I'm fat because of a slow metabolism.

It's true when your thyroid isn't functioning properly it can slow your metabolism and bring your fat loss to a halt. However most people that believe they have a slow metabolism really don't. Instead what they have is a need to jumpstart the body with a combination of good nutrition and aerobic exercise. It's a simple as a 15 minute brisk walk.

Myth #4 – It's possible to keep the weight off even with a fad diet.

If you want to quickly lose 10 pounds a fad diet will certainly allow you to accomplish that quickly. But the research indicates that 80%

of dieters will actually gain the weight back in 5 years. Worse, you'll also lose muscle mass and gain back fat. This might explain why society seems to be getting more overweight as the years go by.

Losing the weight using a diet (even a fad diet) isn't so bad as long as you follow up with healthy lifestyle changes that ensure you keep the weight off.

Myth #5 – I can lose my belly fat doing crunches

Far too many people attempt to get rid of belly fat with no success. What happens is muscle builds under the belly fat and then your belly actually looks bigger. If you want to lose belly fat faster aerobic exercise is the answer – in fact, you'll lose belly fat as much as 10 xs faster with cardiac exercises.

Now that we've uncovered these 5 myths you'll be shedding those extra pounds faster than ever.

CHAPTER 9- DIET AND EXERCISING COMBO TO EXTREME WEIGHT LOSS

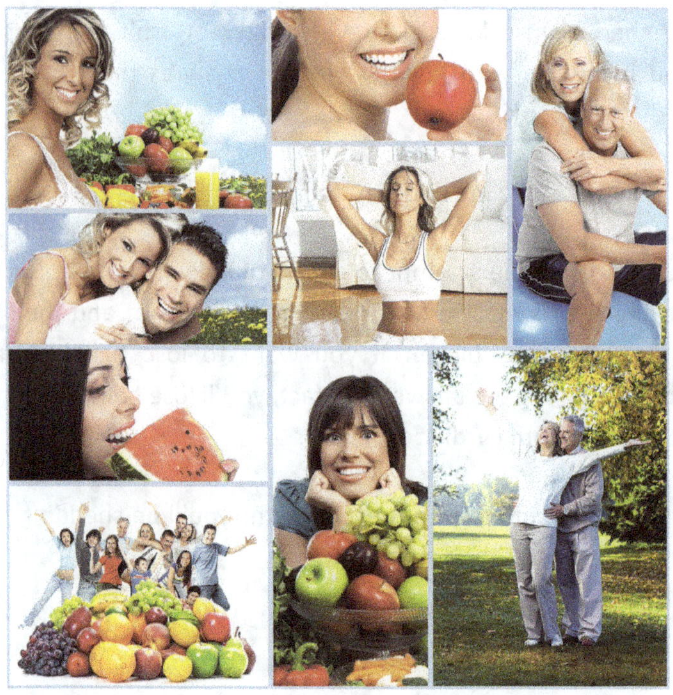

Many, if not all of the weight loss guru's will tell you that exercise and diet must go together. There are many reasons for this, but the main reason is that muscle burns fat faster than fat burns fat. Does that make sense? Many people, like myself, really do not have the time, nor the energy (until you lose the pounds,) nor even the inclination to exercise, but because it helps by leaps and bounds to keep your muscles toned, and burn fat, I started doing isometric exercises that I can do at my desk without ever leaving my chair.

An isometric exercise, in a nutshell, is to tighten your muscles and hold the position for about 10 to 15 seconds, and then let off. It is what is called a "static" exercise, which was all the rage in the 60's when I was growing up. It was popular because it took no special equipment, and you didn't have to join a gym, which were not as popular as they are these days. You choose a group of muscles, let's take for example your stomach muscles, or abs. You can sit at your desk, and tighten those muscles for 15 to 20 seconds, and then relax them for 30 seconds. Do this 3 or 4 times...what we call a "set." You want to make sure you are sitting up in your chair, but the biggest thing to remember is to breathe. A lot of people tend to hold their breath as they are doing the exercises, which can do you more harm than good. Your muscles need the oxygen especially through the exercising stage, so please remember to breathe.

Your arms can be exercised in the same way. Because each arm has several muscle groups, it is important to rotate your hands for each exercise. Let's do one right now as an example. Start by flexing your bicep and forearm, and then gently rotate your hand and wrist back and forth. Can you feel the different muscle groups? Now do the exercise one arm at a time, and with your hand in 3 different positions for 3 separate exercises. Hold them for 15 seconds, remembering to breathe, and then relax them for 30 seconds.

The legs work the same way. Clinching your thigh muscles for 15 seconds, and relax for 30 seconds. Again, 3 sets. Your calf muscles work much in the same way, only you will want to kind of stand on your toes while sitting...for 3 sets. You can, and should to this for your buttocks as well. You will not be "bulking up" during this process, but it will start helping you to tone those muscles, which inevitably will begin your weight loss regimen.

Isometric exercises are not the ideal situation, but will do for our purpose for the time being. As you begin to lose weight, you are going to WANT to do more. You are going to feel that old energy come back...and it is a GREAT feeling. The more you do this, the more weight you will lose, and the more energy you are going to have to possibly venture into doing some walking, or stair stepping, or some other cardio exercises. Believe me, I do NOT like to exercise...but even having the energy to go out and shoot some hoops with the kids, or throwing the baseball or football around, has, like I said before, done worlds for me and my children!

If you would like to see some isometric exercises in action, please click here to see some videos by Dave Hubbard, who is known as America's Fitness Coach. This will explain it much better than I can in words. By the way, the videos are free to watch, and will open in a new window.

While Dave uses barbells in his videos, while they are great, not all of us have access to them. I have found that ANY weight works well, including cans of soup. It gives just a bit more resistance to your workout, which is plenty for our purposes right now.

I am going to repeat this because it bears repeating. We do these exercises to help us burn fat. It will speed your process by leaps and bounds. Honestly, I didn't start using these exercises until I had already lost my initial 20 pounds, which we will be going into in the next phase of the plan.

The thing that triggered my interest in weight loss, was when I quit smoking. I had gained an incredible amount of weight, for me anyway...and I wanted to do something about it. It was getting difficult for me to breathe, I had absolutely no energy, plus the fact that I was getting tired of lying on the bed to fasten my pants. Does any of this sound familiar to you? It was time for a change of some sort, and so I recollected an article that I had read about the benefits of green tea.

This was the catalyst for my success. I replaced my morning coffee with green tea. It was no easy task, as I love my coffee, but I immediately started feeling better. I didn't get my usual morning jitters from too much caffeine, and I seemed to have a bit more energy. I thought that it just might have been in my mind, but it was, in fact, doing something positive to my body.

The following pages will describe exactly what I did to lose this weight, and have been able to keep it off, which has been a huge struggle for many...including myself.

Aside from drinking green tea, my eating habits changed as well, but only for the first 2 weeks. This may be the time that you may have problems also. I usually didn't eat breakfast because I felt I didn't have time. I started to make time to fix myself a little breakfast, which normally consisted of oatmeal and a slice of toast, which filled me up perfectly until lunch. If it wasn't oatmeal, it was a bowl of raisin bran or shredded wheat. I enjoy all 3, and was happy to have a change of scene once in awhile. Eating the same thing day in and day out gets monotonous, and I really wanted to get those pounds off, so the variety was welcomed. The key here is to not let yourself get bored with what you eat. Eggs once or twice a week isn't a bad thing either, at least it wasn't in my case. The importance of breakfast should not be overlooked. You need to EAT to lose weight, believe it or not. If I got hungry between lunch and dinner, I would grab an apple or a banana. I was not willing to clog myself up with any other kinds of things for a snack.

The trick here is to NOT let yourself get hungry. You MUST eat to keep up your metabolism. The diets where you starve yourself can do real damage to your body. Your body will actually cannibalize itself, by stealing essential nutrients from your organs and muscles, to satisfy its requirements in less important areas. You may lose weight, but most times you will gain it back in a very short period...AND it is bad for the rest of your body, especially your organs like the heart and brain.

Snacks between meals are important, as long as it's the right things to eat. Like I said, fresh fruit, (not canned,) and fresh vegetables are the best. I don't think I have to say this, but cookies, candy, and the like will only slow your progress.

Please remember all the way through this guide, that this is exactly what I did to lose 40+ pounds and 4 inches off my waist. I am not pushing any one specific brand of anything here. I buy the cheap stuff...whatever it is. Brand names are fine, if you can afford them and it makes you feel better thinking you are buying a better product, but I have found that the store brands work just as well as the brand names. The only exception to this is that I use the One-A-Day vitamins, and the reasoning behind this is that they have come out with an age specific supplement that is blended to meet the requirements of us older folks. The other supplements I take are, Vitamin C, B Complex, Calcium, Vitamin D, and Vitamin E.

The other "rascal" we have is fast food. NO diet has any chance at all if you continue to stop by McDonalds or Burger King for a "snack". If you are serious about losing weight, fast food joints should go away from your life. When you have completed your goal, give thanks and go treat yourself to a big-mac. You've earned that right, but don't make it a habit.

Coffee vs. Tea

I used to be a hard core coffee drinker. Nobody could have possibly loved their coffee more than I. (I also loved alcohol, but that's another story.) I always thought that if I were to give up anything in my life, it would be anything but my coffee. Therefore, it was the law of the land...or in my house anyway. I wanted to put it in the Bill of Rights, or maybe even the 11th commandment...thou shalt not let me run out of coffee.

I had no idea that coffee was actually hindering my weight loss goals. Again, I didn't find this out until I was curious one day last week and looked it up. This was long after I started losing the pounds.

I want to include this article by James Bowden, which helps explain the affects of coffee on your body.

I myself have had my battles with Starbucks. It's a difficult habit to break (though after writing this column, I'm going to give it a try). I can tell you this, though, both from my experience and from that of others: When you break the coffee habit, you will feel your own power and energy and be in touch with your own natural energetic rhythms. You may even find that a caffeine-free existence is a great boost to your weight-loss efforts.

Although I am not be ready to say that something as basic to American life as coffee is a "drug," we can certainly say that it has drug-like properties:

• It's addictive.

• It's a stimulant.

• It alters mood.

And -- it's not good for weight loss.

There are two basic reasons coffee is a problem for the person trying to lose weight. (It's no bargain for the person who isn't either, by the way). The first reason is psychological, the second physiological.

Psychological

Coffee fits neatly into the receptors for a brain chemical known as adenosine, which is partly responsible for calming you down. By interrupting the activity of adenosine, coffee makes you feel awake and wired. You may think that's a good thing, but consider that virtually every study of PMS has implicated caffeine as a major culprit. The added stimulation and nervousness from the coffee makes you feel edgy at exactly the time that feeling calm would be a blessing. And the blood sugar fluctuations it produces contributes enormously to cravings.

Coffee is socially connected to rituals that involve eating. Many of these eating rituals, in turn, are connected to snacks and breaks, fast-food breakfasts and desserts. (Notice that the first beverage you think of when asked what you want with your "Dunkin' Donuts" is not green tea or water.)

Physiological

Coffee stimulates the adrenals, the glands responsible for stress hormones. The constant assault on these poor glands, from coffee, sugar, stress and daily life, can ultimately lead to a condition known as adrenal exhaustion.

Coffee plays havoc with your blood sugar. The body treats a coffee jolt as a "stress response" much like the adrenals shooting a jolt of adrenaline into the system. This adrenaline response was a survival mechanism for our caveman ancestors; it signaled danger from a woolly mammoth and told the body to prepare for fight or flight. It signaled the body to release sugar into the blood, to be used as fuel for the muscles (which would be either clubbing that mammoth or climbing the nearest tree). But nowadays, it just signals the release of sugar. With no ensuing flight or flight, the sugar signals a release of insulin, and before you know it, after a couple of hours of jitteriness, your blood sugar is in the toilet, and you're crashing and burning and reaching for ... guess what? I'll give you a hint: It's not Brussels sprouts and steak.

Coffee also increases urinary secretion of important minerals such as magnesium, potassium and sodium and uses up a fair amount of vitamin B1. Not only that, the coffee plant itself is a virtual repository for toxins such as pesticides and other harmful chemicals. (If you still insist on drinking it after reading this article, consider buying organic). And it can raise blood pressure and interfere with sleep.

Although in the short run it may suppress appetite, over the course of a day most people find it stimulates cravings more than suppresses them.

One of the best reasons to give up coffee comes from my colleague, Dr. Barry Sears, who points out that if you are "running on empty," getting your "energy" from artificial stimulants like caffeine, you never really get to understand the effect your food is having on you. You never know whether your food is producing energy and alertness or tiredness and fatigue. You're masking the effects of your eating style with an overpowering stimulant. And that's keeping you from valuable knowledge about what foods work for you and what foods you ought to stay away from.

There is a myth that coffee and green tea have the same amount of calories. Nothing could be further from the truth.

The average cup of coffee can have anywhere from 80-175 mg of caffeine, depending on the method of preparation. By comparison, the average cup of green tea has about 25-30mg of caffeine.

Furthermore, green tea has a number of health benefits (preventing cancer, battling diabetes, fighting cholesterol, boosting the immune system...) and it is recommended to drink 4-5 cups each day to reap the full benefits. According to researchers, it's safe to drink up 10 cups of green tea a day.

In extreme amounts, the high amounts of polyphenols can cause liver or kidney damage--green tea *supplements* can have dangerously high levels.

However, some people are very sensitive to caffeine; if you do find yourself feeling jittery or having heart palpitations, try cutting back on the tea. Also, tea is a diuretic, which increases urination. I'd say that, aside from frequent bathroom breaks, you should be fine.

(Incidentally, green tea is best brewed at 180 degrees F, which is just under a boil. If you brew your tea at too high a temperature, you lose a lot of the health benefits. It also tastes better at a lower temp.)

There is some controversy about women drinking green tea while pregnant, or wanting to become pregnant. PLEASE CONSULT YOUR DOCTOR before you go off and do this on your own. Having a healthy baby is, by far, more important than any diet. There is time to lose the pounds after the baby is born!

Okay...here we go! I am now going to explain exactly what my daily routine consists of to lose 40+ pounds and 4 inches off of my waistline while sitting on my duff!

Chapter 10- The Plan to Extreme Weight Loss

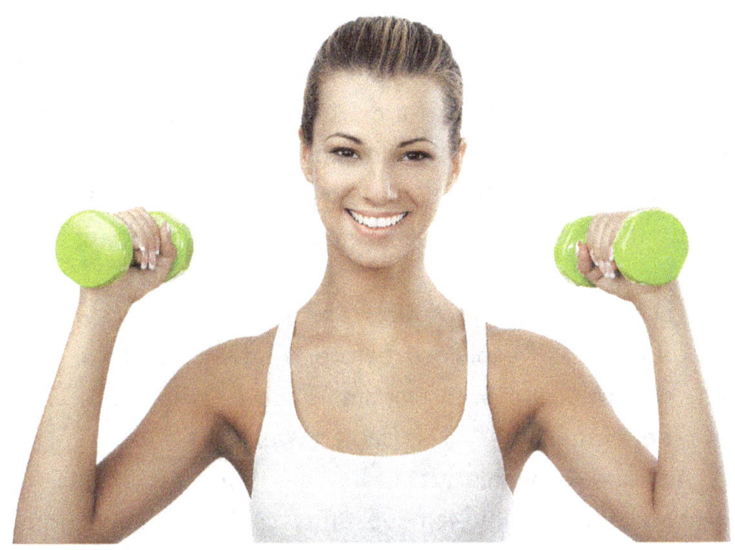

For the first 1 or 2 weeks, this may be difficult for you. We are essentially shrinking our stomachs, and replacing bad habits with good habits. Do not skip breakfast! Remember, our body needs the fuel to carry on through the day.

I wake up every morning at 4 am. This is not necessary for you to do, it's just what my body clock is used to. When I get up, my green tea is waiting for me. I use my coffee maker to brew my tea, and I make a full pot that will last me all day. 3 cups in the morning, and the rest for iced tea during the day. I might decide, instead, to have it hot, so I just stick it in the microwave. I use 6 teabags for a full, 12 cup pot. You may use more, or less, depending on your particular taste, but remember that while the tea sits, it will get darker and stronger. Since it is naturally sweet, I use no sugar, but if you have to sweeten it, use a sugar substitute. I really dislike the chemicals used for the sugar substitute, so I avoid them...again, personal preference.

I said earlier that I buy the cheap brands, and that includes my tea. I use my store brand of green tea. It is cheaper, and as far as I can tell, it doesn't make a difference.

Remember, I sit at my computer for a large part of the day, so while I am sitting there, taking a small break, I do my isometric exercises. Sometimes while I am working I do it. It depends on what part of the body I am working on. It is pretty difficult to work on your arm muscles while typing, so I have to take a break to do those, but the legs and buttocks exercises are pretty easy to do.

After I get the kids off to school, I take a break from my work and have breakfast. As I explained before, a bowl of oatmeal, (heart healthy,) which I cook with cinnamon and a teaspoon of vanilla. YUM! I top it off with 2% milk, (same taste, less fat,) and 1 slice of toast. Any kind of whole grain is great! If you can't handle the thought of oatmeal, you can substitute cold cereal...but nothing with sugar. Eggs with 1 slice of toast may also be used. The point here is to start off your day right, and have some kind of breakfast. If not, your body is in starvation mode, and therefore starts to store fat because it thinks you are trying to starve it. The body is wonderful that way. It is self-preservation at its best.

One thing I would like to add to this. I use real butter only. I did some research a few years back about the benefits of margarine for a healthier lifestyle. I was shocked to find out that margarine is actually only 1 molecule away from plastic. Your body gets confused with chemicals. The body knows how to break down butter...so I haven't touched margarine since.

I know that you may think it crazy that I am supporting dairy and bread for our purposes, but this works. The trick is not to go overboard. One slice of bread per meal is not going to hurt a thing.

2 to 3 hours after breakfast, grab yourself an apple, banana, a carrot, whatever you have that is fresh and wholesome. This is to satisfy any craving you may have at this point. It is not lunch...so don't worry.

For lunch, I make myself a can of soup, normally water based, and half a sandwich. I either have ham, turkey, or chicken, and use mayo or miracle whip, (my preference,) on a slice of bread. Whatever bread you see fit is fine. Don't get stuck giving yourself something that you can't tolerate. If you prefer white bread, go for it. I prefer the whole grain breads, but I don't know that it actually makes that much of a difference. I sometimes treat myself with a peanut butter sandwich, but not often. There's a lot of sugar in peanut butter, but hey, again it is half a sandwich. Just don't go overboard and put half an inch of peanut butter on your bread. It defeats the whole purpose.

If I get hungry again a couple of hours later, you guessed it, another piece of fruit. A glass of green tea, hot or cold, is also in order.

Dinner time for my family is at about 6pm. I have another cup of green tea about a half hour before mealtime. This helps raise my metabolic rate to where I am not as hungry as I had been in the past. (This is according to my research. I was curious to learn why I was dropping so much weight.) For the first 2 weeks I ate very little pasta, and no fried foods at all. Those are the only 2 things I gave up over the 2 week period. Instead, I would eat sensibly. I started off with a small salad with just a small amount of dressing, (just enough to flavor it slightly,) and a meat of some kind, like baked chicken or a steak. It was satisfying for my taste buds, and I felt full. I no longer heaped my plate with mashed potatoes and gravy, or whatever the starch was that night. I just held off, and realized that it didn't need that much food to feel satisfied.

After 2 weeks of eating this way, I was feeling better than I had in years. I had lost about 10 pounds during this first 2 weeks, and I was hungry for more. I didn't want to be fat any more, and knew that I had stumbled upon the solution to get me back into shape.

I was amazed at how simple it actually was. I was losing weight, and not suffering. I was eating pretty much what I had been before, only in smaller amounts, and I was happy. I decided to take my "experiment" to the next level. My stomach either shrunk, or my metabolism changed, or something...but I no longer needed, nor wanted, vast amounts of food. I like the feeling of comfortable instead of GORGED!

Since all of this was making sense to me now, I continued down that same path, only now I was eating anything the family had. I missed my pasta, and my pizza...so, I started eating those again as well. I continued with my green tea, and ate half as much as I used to. As an example, before all this started, I would eat a whole pizza in one sitting. I still think I could if I tried, but why? I am very comfortable eating half, and saving the other half for my lunch the next day. I am full...and that is what my body wants. My stomach doesn't want any more food, so why would I continue to stuff it? It would only make me feel miserable.

Instead of a plate mounded with spaghetti, I chose to eat half that amount. Again, because of the combination of green tea before dinner, and my smaller stomach, I didn't need any more than what I had dished up for myself. Many times I didn't even finish what I had in front of me. THAT is another problem. We are taught from an early age to finish what is on our plates. If we follow that logic, we need to put less food on there in the first place. Don't let your taste buds tell you that you have to have more, when your stomach is telling you otherwise. It is not healthy, and you will eventually get back into the trap of forcing your stomach to grow again. Little by little, we will keep expanding our stomach to its former size...and we don't want that to happen...right?

That is the only thing I did in my weight loss strategy, and I am continuing to lose weight as we speak. Continuing with my green tea, eating healthier without becoming fanatical about it, and at this point, eating what I want...only in smaller portions.

You may have noticed that I have not said anything about calories so far, so let's chat about that for a bit.

A calorie is a unit of energy. We will not go into the scientific mumbo-jumbo to explain everything it is and does. Human beings need energy to survive -- to breathe, move, and pump blood -- and they acquire this energy from food. The number of calories in a food is a measure of how much potential energy that food possesses. A gram of carbohydrates has 4 calories, a gram of protein has 4 calories and a gram of fat has 9 calories. Foods are a compilation of these three building blocks. So if you know how many carbohydrates, fats and proteins are in any given food, you know how many calories, or how much energy, that food contains.

It seems that every food in the grocery store has the amount of calories on the label. It seems that the normal intake of calories they figure for a person is about 2,000 calories per day. This varies from person to person, however. A lot depends on how active your lifestyle is. A person like me, (relatively inactive because I spend most days planted in front of a computer) needs fewer calories than an active person who slings heavy boxes all day long.

About the Author

Linda Davis is a well-known nutritionist and a certified holistic instructor. She admits that she is not perfect and that she still considers herself as someone who needs to be improved when it comes to staying fit at all times. According to Linda, there are a lot of temptations that she encounters on a daily basis that are against her diet plan and diet regimen.

This book is not only a guide for you to get that body and lifestyle that you've been wanting but also for her Linda as well. Linda has small gym in Virginia where she lives with her family.

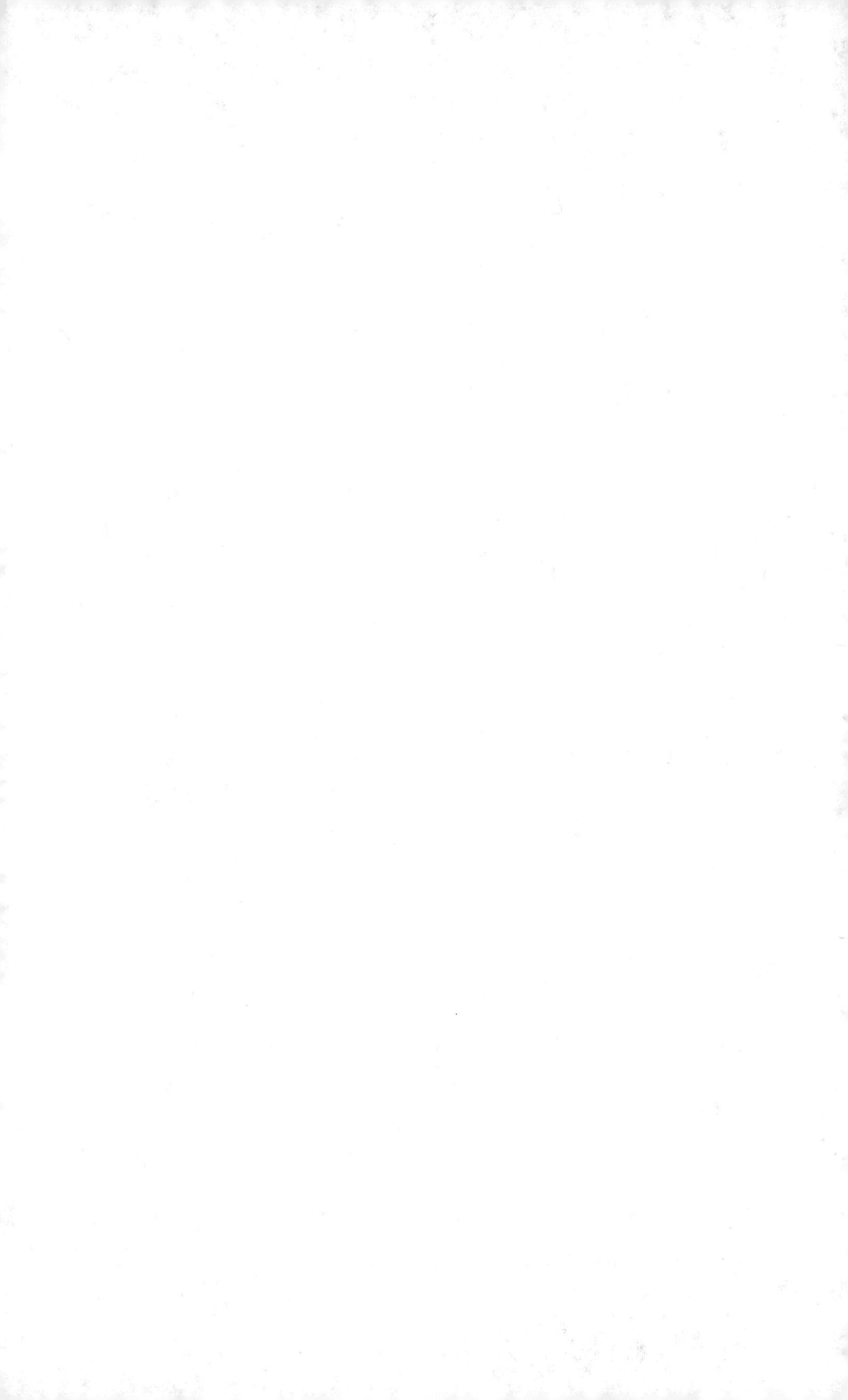